PERIOD SEX

Exploring the Depths of Desire During Your Cycle

Helene Yorke

Table of Contents

Introduction

Since Emily and Alex had been together for so long, their bond was solid and based on trust. They were both curious and open-minded, so when the subject of period sex came up in a late-night discussion.

They spoke about their emotions and limitations to make sure they were both at ease. They prepared the scene for an intimate encounter the next time Emily's period came.

A new level of intimacy grew as they accepted their desires. They were more intimate than ever because of the increased sensitivity and vulnerability.

The pleasure they enjoyed gave Emily a break from her period symptoms. Alex was in awe of the organic lubrication that enhanced their enjoyment.

But more than simply the physical interactions contributed to their closer friendship.

Their openness to discussing their wants and desires in frank dialogues strengthened their emotional closeness.

Period sex came to represent their unshakable love and trust. The exploration had not only been enjoyable for Emily and Alex, but it had also improved their bond.

It served as a reminder that facing the unknown together may result in lovely and significant discoveries and strengthen a bond that would last.

Chapter One

Unveiling The Taboo Surrounding Period Sex

Few issues in the domain of human experience are as shrouded in secret and whispers as period sex.

Despite being a normal part of life for half of the world's population, talks regarding participating in sexual activity during menstruation typically remain cloaked in cultural misconceptions, misunderstandings, and apprehensions.

The mere notion of period sex may elicit a wide range of emotions, including fascination, repulsion, discomfort, and curiosity.

This taboo around period sex has significant historical, cultural, and sociological origins.

Menstruation has long been associated with stories that combine ideas of impurity, secrecy, and shame. These stories have contributed to the topic's cautious quiet.

However, at a time characterized by the goal of openness and education, it is imperative to dispel myths regarding period sex, dispel misinformation, and arm people with factual knowledge.

The advantages, drawbacks, dangers to unborn children, and advice related to period sex openly and sympathetically, and other related subjects will be discussed, working to dispel the discomfort and myths that have clouded this normal aspect of human connection.

Continue with this enlightening book as we shed light on the facts, dispel misconceptions, and promote an honest discussion about period sex.

Let knowledge eliminate the stigma so that we may approach this subject with curiosity, empathy, and the freedom to choose how we want to feel about our bodies, our relationships, and our desires.

Chapter Two

The Advantages of Period Sex

Period sex, which is sometimes veiled in secrecy and myths, has several advantages beyond what is generally thought to be forbidden.

It's crucial to investigate and comprehend the benefits that period sex may provide in a society when frank discussions about sexual health are gaining traction.

Let's explore these advantages, highlighting the often-overlooked facets of human connection and well-being.

A. Physical and Emotional Intimacy

The confluence of physical and emotional closeness emerges as an appealing aspect among the rumors and misconceptions that often surround the subject of period sex.

Period sex is a chance to explore and strengthen the tie between lovers on both a physical and emotional level in a society where sincere connections are valued.

Physical intimacy is a must. Menstruating while having sex may be an indication of a connection that goes beyond the confines of the menstrual cycle.

As couples negotiate a normal biological process together, the act itself calls for a higher degree of comfort, trust, and vulnerability.

A feeling of intimacy and connection that goes beyond physical sensations may be created by the desire to hug each other's bodies at this time.

Let's look at the surprising ways that menstruation may increase both physical desire and sensuous sensations:

Emotional Bonding: A greater emotional connection between lovers might result from sharing the period sex experience. The willingness to share private moments at a time when one could feel more exposed highlights the degree of trust and understanding in the partnership. A stronger feeling of cooperation and more honest communication might result from this shared experience.

Mutual Acceptance: Period sex gives people the chance to accept one another completely, including the physiological traits that make us human. Partners show a degree of compassion and love that is beyond cultural standards and expectations by tolerating and participating in activities during menstruation.

Increased Trust: Period sex involves open communication and permission from both parties. Openly addressing preferences, limits, and wants fosters a climate of respect and trust, which improves the relationship's overall quality.

Improved Connection: Period sex fosters a special feeling of connection that may be hard to reproduce in other settings due to the merging of physical pleasure and emotional intimacy. The act takes on the form of a shared trip that the two couples start together, strengthening their bond.

A certain level of comprehension, open communication, and a willingness to accept closeness outside of social norms are necessary for navigating the world of period sex.

Couples build the basis for a deeper relationship that recognizes and appreciates the complexities of human nature as they explore the physical and emotional aspects of this experience.

Period sex becomes a tribute to the wonder of human connection in all of its forms by developing an atmosphere of trust, permission, and shared vulnerability.

B. Boosted Libido and Sensitivity

An unanticipated phenomenon, an increase in desire and sensitivity, often occurs in the world of period sex.

This aspect sheds light on a degree of pleasure that defies preconceptions among the misunderstandings and hesitations that surround this subject.

Let's look at the surprising ways that menstruation may boost libido and sensitivity:

Increased Sensitivity: Many people claim that their menstrual cycle makes them more sensitive. Greater awareness of bodily feelings may result from the increased blood flow to the pelvic region. This may result in a more intense feeling of touch, resulting in more sexual pleasure.

Stimulation that Arouses: Arousal levels may be greater during menstruation due to the increased blood flow to the pelvic area. This physical reaction may intensify the feelings felt during sexual activity, making it more enjoyable for both participants.

Increasing Orgasms: Increased sensitivity and excitement can cause orgasms to become more intense. Stronger and more pleasurable climaxes may result from the body's increased physiological reactions, providing a rare chance for sexual exploration.

Relationship between Partners: Menstruation-related sensitivity and heightened desire may lead to a feeling of adventure and exploration between lovers. Couples might learn new methods to enjoy closeness and pleasure by having sexual activity during this period, building a closer bond.

Difficult Presumptions: The feeling of increased libido and sensitivity challenges the idea that menstruation cycles innately reduce sexual desire. This discovery inspires people to listen to their bodies and question cultural myths that may not be true to their personal experiences.

Menstruation may increase certain people's desire and sensitivity, which highlights the richness and variety of human sexuality. Couples may start on a voyage of discovery and pleasure, changing their concept of intimacy, by embracing this aspect of period sex.

Accepting the possibility of greater pleasure and connection during menstruation may result in a more gratifying and powerful experience for all individuals involved as talks about sexual health become more open and inclusive.

C. Menstrual Pain Relief

A surprising advantage emerges among the difficulties of menstruation: possible pain reduction. Although it may seem contradictory to engage in sexual activity at this time, endorphin release and the physiological reactions brought on by excitement may help to lessen menstrual pain.

Let's explore how period sex might be a surprisingly effective method of reducing menstruation discomfort:

Endorphin: A natural pain reliever sometimes referred to be the body's natural painkillers, are released as a result of sexual activity. Endorphins are neurochemicals that provide pleasurable emotions and function as analgesics, which help to lessen pain perceptions.

Relaxation of Muscles: Muscle relaxation may occur throughout the body, including the pelvic area, as a result of sexual excitement and activity. The alleviation from cramps and tension brought on by this relaxation might aid women who are experiencing menstruation discomfort.

Enhanced Blood Flow: Sexual activity boosts blood flow to the pelvic region, which may lessen the pain brought on by menstrual cramps. Increased circulation may help to relieve pain and relax tight muscles.

Distraction Effect: Menstrual discomfort may be diverted by engaging in exciting and rewarding activities, such as sexual engagement. Temporary alleviation may be obtained by diverting the brain's attention away from pain and toward pleasant feelings.

Personalized Experience: Depending on the individual, period sex may have different impacts on menstrual discomfort. While some people could feel a lot better, others might not notice much of a change. It's crucial to be truthful with your spouse and pay attention to your body's signals.

While there isn't a one-size-fits-all approach to menstruation pain relief, period sex does emphasize the complex ways in which our bodies react to closeness and pleasure.

By accepting the potential that sexual activity might relieve discomfort, people pave the way for a more comprehensive approach to menstrual health.

Awareness of the many advantages of period sex helps to a more thorough awareness of our bodies and their possibilities for pleasure and comfort as discussions about sexual health and wellbeing continue to develop.

D.   Improved   Mood   and Relaxation

An unexpected source of comfort comes during menstrual periods when mood swings and emotional variations might throw a shadow enhanced mood and relaxation via period sex.

Contrary to popular belief, sexual activity during this period might cause hormonal reactions that support a higher feeling of well-being and emotional equilibrium.

Let's look at how period sex may act as a bridge to more mellow feelings.

Oxytocin Release: The "love hormone" or "cuddle hormone," oxytocin, is released in response to sexual intercourse. Bonding, relaxation, and emotional connection are promoted by oxytocin. The spike in oxytocin may reduce mood swings and promote emotional stability and satisfaction.

Stress Reduction: Stress and anxiety may be reduced by partaking in enjoyable activities like sexual intercourse. Period sex stimulates the brain's reward system, which lowers stress levels via the physical and mental pleasure it brings.

Distracting Oneself from Uncomfort: Sexual activity's beneficial side effects might serve as a distraction from menstruation pain. In times of physical distress, pleasant feelings, and emotional connection may take the place of painful ones, providing a welcome diversion.

Sleep Promotion: During sexual activity, oxytocin and other hormones are released, which may promote relaxation and a greater feeling of well-being. This may result in better sleep, which has a favorable effect on mood and emotional well-being in general.

Improvement of Emotional Wellness: Accepting period sex challenges society's standards and gives people the ability to make decisions in line with their preferences and level of comfort.

This empowerment may support improved mental health and self-esteem, encouraging a more positive perspective on one's appearance and choices. People have access to a level of emotional solace and connection during period sex that defies expectations.

This newly discovered viewpoint challenges prejudices and motivates people to put their emotional well-being first, making wise decisions that honor both pleasure and emotional balance.

Chapter Three

Side Effects and Concerns: Navigating the Terrain of Period Sex

It's important to be aware of any possible negative impacts and worries people may have when we discuss the topic of period sex. While period sex has many advantages, there are a few things to keep in mind.

Let's explore these elements in further detail to illuminate the complex context of this private decision.

A. Messiness and Hygiene

One of the main issues that often come up while exploring the world of period sex is the possibility of messiness and its effect on cleanliness.

While these worries are real, they may be efficiently dealt with by being prepared, having open communication, and approaching intimacy with awareness.

Let's look at how to have period sex while putting comfort and cleanliness first.

Communication is Key: Have an honest discussion with your spouse before having period sex. Together, go through any worries you may have about messiness. Sharing your thoughts, preferences, and any limits may help to establish a comfortable environment where both parties can take pleasure in the interaction.

Select the Right Environment: Decide on an environment where you are both at ease and comfortable. Use dark blankets or towels to help hide any stains as much as possible. You may relax and concentrate on the connection by creating a space that is accommodating of possible messiness.

Hygiene Preparations: Both parties may follow meticulous hygiene procedures before having sexual activity. Menstrual fluid may be reduced by showering or cleaning the vaginal region. A water-based lubricant may reduce friction and improve comfort.

Menstrual Supplies: Menstrual hygiene supplies should be kept nearby and simple to get. Before participating in sexual activity, if you'd like, you may also use a menstrual cup or sponge that can be covertly inserted.

Towel or Mat: You may assist by limiting any possible mess and allay concerns about ruining bedding by placing a towel or waterproof mat underneath you. This sensible answer might help make the experience more carefree and pleasurable. Remember that menstruation fluid is a normal component of the human body and embraces openness.

Adopt an accepting and open mindset toward yourself as well as your relationship. This viewpoint might make the situation more inviting and put both parties at ease.

A cooperative and thoughtful approach is necessary to navigate the messiness and hygiene issues that might arise during period sex.

You may establish an environment where intimacy can grow while maintaining comfort and hygiene by placing a priority on open communication, creating the ideal mood, and taking practical precautions.

Period sex ultimately turns into a chance for mutual vulnerability, comprehension, and connection, enabling you and your partner to travel this sensitive trip with caution and respect.

B. Potential Discomfort

It's crucial to acknowledge the possibility of discomfort that some people may feel as we explore the world of period sex. Sexual activity during a menstrual period may intensify a variety of bodily sensations that might be brought on by the cycle.

However, period sex may be handled in a manner that promotes comfort and connection for both participants with conversation, understanding, and a commitment to prioritize well-being.

Open Communication: Have an honest discussion with your spouse before having period sex. If you have any worries or discomfort, let your partner know, and urge them to do the same. Making room for open communication may aid both parties in navigating the situation with empathy and understanding.

Listen to Your Body: Pay great attention to the messages and feelings coming from your body. If you're uncomfortable, let your partner know and think about other types of closeness that put your comfort first. Keep in mind that obtaining permission is a continuous process, so put your comfort first at all times.

Select Pleasant Positions: Try out various sexual positions to see which ones are most pleasant for both parties. While certain postures may make you feel more uncomfortable, others could do the opposite. To ensure a great experience, communication and flexibility are essential.

Focus on Emotional Connection: If physical pain is an issue, think about putting your attention on your emotional connection and closeness. Activities that promote emotional intimacy, like kissing, hugging, or sharing tender moments, may help couples stay connected without endangering their well-being.

Be Patient and Understanding: Every person's experience with periods is different, and they may cause a variety of bodily feelings. Be tolerant and patient with yourself as well as your lover. It's crucial that you put one another's comfort and well-being first.

Respect and empathy are necessary while navigating possible discomfort during period sex. Couples may make sure the experience is good for both parties by putting open communication, active consent, and dedication to each other's well-being first.

It's important to customize the experience so that it reflects your comfort level and personal preferences since intimacy is a journey that encompasses both physical and emotional connections.

C. Prioritizing Safe Practices to Reduce Infection Risk

The possible danger of infection should be considered while thinking about period sex. Sexual activity during menstruation might change the environment in the vagina, which could make it more likely for germs to thrive there and cause an infection.

However, the danger may be reduced with the right safety measures and cleanliness habits.

Let's look at how to put safety first while maintaining intimacy when on your period.

Maintain Cleanliness: It's critical to practice meticulous cleanliness both before and after sexual activity. It is recommended that both spouses cleanse their genitalia with water and gentle, unscented soap. This reduces the amount of microorganisms present and keeps the environment clean.

Use Protection: Using protection may provide a barrier that lowers the chance of infection. Examples include the use of condoms. In addition to preventing the transmission of STIs, condoms also aid in limiting the spread of new germs into the vaginal environment.

Avoid Using Shared Objects: Avoid putting any items into the vaginal region that have come into touch with menstruation fluid. These things might be fingers, sex toys, or something else. If you decide to utilize sex toys, make sure to wash and sterilize them both before and after each usage.

Watch for Changes: Pay close attention to any changes in the health of your vagina, such as odd discharge, odor, or pain. Consult a healthcare provider if you have any unusual symptoms as a result of period sex.

Urinate After Sex: Urinating helps remove germs from the urethra, lowering the risk of urinary tract infections (UTIs). The maintenance of urinary tract health is made more vital by this procedure following period sex.

Menstrual Tools: Tools such as tampons or menstrual cups, should be kept clean. Also, make sure they are inserted correctly. Regularly changing these items and practicing good cleanliness may help stop the spread of new microorganisms.

Prioritize Communication: Talk to your spouse honestly about any worries or discomfort you may be experiencing. It is essential to have respect for one another's beliefs and devotion to their safety and well-being.

The risk of infection connected with period sex may be considerably decreased by using safe procedures and maintaining adequate cleanliness.

A happy and secure personal encounter is facilitated by putting an emphasis on open communication, employing protection, and paying attention to your body's cues.

The secret is to approach period sex with caution and regard for the well-being of both parties, making sure that enjoyment and safety go hand in hand.

D. Impact on Sexual Desire

Exploring the effects of period sex on sexual desire is one thing to keep in mind. Individual preferences for sexual activity may change as a result of mood, physical feelings, and hormonal changes brought on by menstrual cycles.

Partners may manage the ebb and flow of desire during menstruation by being aware of these variations and addressing them with open dialogue and understanding.

Open and Honest Conversation: This is essential for addressing changes in sexual desire. Encourage your spouse to express their thoughts and preferences by doing the same. This fosters an atmosphere where both people feel comfortable and able to communicate their aspirations.

Respect Individual Preferences: Awareness of the individuality of each person's menstrual cycle experience. While some people may sense a drop in sexual desire during their periods, others may experience an increase. Respect one another's choices and put mutual agreement first.

Investigate Alternate kinds of Intimacy: If one partner's desire to be intimate decreases during menstruation, take into account investigating alternate kinds of intimacy. Maintaining emotional intimacy may be facilitated by actions like snuggling, kissing, and sharing private moments without engaging in penetrative intercourse.

Embrace Flexibility: It's normal for sexual desire to fluctuate throughout menstruation. Be adaptable and understanding of each other's needs and emotions. Keep in mind that your mental bond is equally as important as your physical closeness.

Experiment with Timing: If one partner experiences a decline in sexual desire during the menstrual cycle's peak, you may want to think about having sex on days when your period isn't as painful. The desires of both couples may be accommodated with this flexibility.

Prioritize Emotional Connection: Sharing ideas and emotions and other forms of emotional closeness may help you stay connected even when your partner's sexual desire isn't as strong. An emotionally pleasant and balanced relationship benefits from intimacy.

Sensitivity, empathy, and mutual understanding are required to navigate the effects of menstrual periods on sexual desire. You may establish an atmosphere where intimacy is governed by agreement and mutual respect by encouraging a place where both partners can communicate their thoughts and preferences without fear of judgment.

In the end, the secret is to respect one another's journeys and keep a bond that endures despite the regular ups and downs of desire.

Chapter Four

Pregnancy Risks and Considerations

When talking about period sex, it's crucial to bring out the possible pregnancy risks and issues connected to having sex while menstruating.

Although there is often a lesser chance of conception at this time, it is important to be aware of the variables that might affect fertility.

Individuals and couples may take action that is in line with their reproductive objectives by comprehending the complexity of fertility windows and the diversity of menstrual cycles.

Chances of Pregnancy During Menstruation: Although there are fewer opportunities to become pregnant during menstruation than at other points in the cycle, it is still possible. Sperm may remain viable in the reproductive system for many days, and early ovulation, which can sometimes happen soon after menstruation finishes, increases the chance of pregnancy.

Variability of Menstrual Cycle Durations: Menstrual cycle durations might vary from person to person. Ovulation may happen closer to the end of the menstrual period in some people's shorter cycles. Due to this variation, the fertile window for some people may coincide with menstruation or the days immediately after.

Sperm Survival and Fertility Window: Sperm may live for up to five days within the female reproductive system, according. There is a chance that sperm will fertilize an egg if ovulation takes place within a few days after the end of menstruation. This underlines how crucial it is to understand your cycle and any possible connections between menstruation and fertility.

Use of Protection: It is advised to use protection, such as condoms or other types of contraception if preventing pregnancy is a top goal. In addition to serving as a barrier against conception, condoms also shield users against STIs, which are always a possibility regardless of the stage of the menstrual cycle.

Monitoring and Information: Understanding your menstrual cycle is crucial. Consider charting your cycle using techniques like measuring cervical mucus consistency or basal body temperature if you want to have period sex while reducing the chance of becoming pregnant.

Consult a Healthcare Professional: A healthcare professional or a reproductive health specialist may provide individualized advice based on your unique situation if you have particular questions regarding pregnancy risks and fertility.

Individuals and couples may make decisions that are in line with their reproductive objectives when they are informed about the complexities of fertility and pregnancy risks during menstruation.

Even while period sex may provide special chances for connection, it's crucial to make judgments that balance sexual enjoyment and reproductive health.

You may navigate the world of period sex with confidence and clarity by combining education, communication, and appropriate behaviors.

Chapter Five

Tips for Enjoyable and Safe Period Sex

Navigating Pleasure and Well-Being

When addressed with care, communication, and an emphasis on well-being, period sex may be a rewarding and personal experience.

You may create a setting where enjoyment, safety, and respect are given priority by implementing these suggestions into your private times.

Open and Honest Communication: Communication with your partner is the cornerstone of a successful relationship. Talk about your preferences, personal limits, and any worries you may have regarding period sex. Both parties may feel heard and understood when a secure environment is created for conversation.

Use of Protection: Using protection is essential if you are not actively attempting to conceive. In addition to protecting against pregnancy, condoms also help lower the risk of STIs. Verify any additional methods of birth control you use to support your reproductive objectives.

Try Different Positions: The best positions and methods to use is try different positions that are fun and comfortable for both parties. While menstruating, certain postures could be more suited than others. Prioritize postures that reduce pain and enable simple cleaning, if needed.

Maintaining Hygiene and Cleanliness: Before participating in sexual intercourse, both parties should exercise strict hygiene. This involves rinsing the genital region with water and mild, unscented soap. Having access to menstrual hygiene products may help ensure a clean and pleasant period.

Pay attention to your body's level of comfort: Your comfort and well-being come first. Pay attention to how your body is feeling and let your spouse know if anything is off. It's OK to stop or transition to different types of intimacy that put your comfort first if you ever feel uncomfortable.

Prepare the Environment: To assist control any messiness, think about using dark-colored bedding or towels. It might be easier to relax and concentrate on the experience if you have a specific area for cleaning.

Embrace Emotional Connection: Remember that period sex is a time to connect emotionally as well as experience physical feelings. Accept the intimacy, openness, and shared experiences that lead to emotional connectedness.

Respect Individual Choices: Period sex is an individual choice, and both parties should be at ease with the option. If one partner is not into period sex, accept their decision without pressuring or criticizing them.

By keeping these suggestions in mind, you and your partner may handle period sex with caution, respect, and awareness. You may establish a pleasant and joyful environment where intimacy thrives by placing a high priority on communication, comfort, and well-being.

Chapter Six

When to Seek Medical Advice

Prioritizing Your Health and Well-Being

While many people find period sex to be a natural and joyful aspect of intimacy, there are certain circumstances when getting medical help is crucial to protect your health and well-being.

Pay attention to these warning signs and, if required, think about seeing a doctor.

Unusual Menstrual Cycles: It's a good idea to speak with a healthcare professional if you have irregular menstrual cycles when the time or flow of your periods changes greatly. Cycle irregularities may be a sign of underlying health problems that need care.

Unusual Pain or Discomfort: While some discomfort throughout the menstrual cycle may be natural, intense or unexpected pain should not be disregarded. Consult a healthcare provider if you have severe cramps, pain during sexual activity, or discomfort that greatly limits your ability to carry out your everyday activities.

Health or Infection-Related Concerns: Consult a doctor if you have any worries about the potential for infection or other health issues connected to period sex. A healthcare professional may provide you with individualized advice and solve any queries or worries you might have.

Modifications in Vaginal Discharge: It may indicate an infection or other medical conditions if you observe modifications to your vaginal discharge, such as an odd odor, color, or consistency. Speak with a medical expert for an assessment.

Persistent Symptoms: Consult a healthcare professional for a comprehensive evaluation if you encounter persistent symptoms that are affecting your general well-being, such as exhaustion, mood swings, or changes in your monthly cycles.

Existing Medical Conditions: Discuss your intentions for having period sex with your healthcare practitioner if you have any pre-existing medical illnesses, such as endometriosis, polycystic ovarian syndrome (PCOS), or other reproductive health issues. They can provide advice tailored to your circumstances.

Unanswered Inquiries: Consult a healthcare practitioner for precise and individualized advice if you have any unresolved issues or worries about how period sex could affect your health or particular situations.

It is crucial to put your health and well-being first. Consulting a healthcare professional may provide you clarity and peace of mind if you're uncertain about whether certain features of period sex are safe or appropriate for you.

Keep in mind that healthcare specialists are there to assist you in making choices that are consistent with your general health objectives.

Chapter Seven

Navigating Period Sex with Knowledge and Confidence

Exploring the world of period sex is a rare chance to enhance intimacy, encourage connection, and question sexuality-related social conventions.

You may manage this personal experience with knowledge and confidence by embracing open communication, being aware of your body's rhythms, and placing a high priority on cleanliness and well-being.

We've examined all the facets of period sex in this guide, from the advantages and factors to the possible difficulties and safety measures. We've emphasized how crucial it is to communicate with your partner, how useful it is to utilize protection, and how crucial it is to choose positions and methods that favor comfort.

We've also covered issues like cleanliness, possible pain, and pregnancy dangers, providing advice on how to carefully handle these complexities.

Period sex is a chance to appreciate your body's physiological functions and appreciate the nuanced nature of romantic closeness.

You may establish an atmosphere where both partners feel empowered to make decisions that are in line with their needs and well-being by encouraging open communication, mutual respect, and consent.

The most important thing is that you approach period sex in a manner that is consistent with your choices, beliefs, and health concerns. Keep in mind that each person's experience is unique.

Approach period sex with the understanding, confidence, and respect for your body that it deserves as you set out on this expedition.

Dear Valued Reader,

Wild your imagination, imagine it and make it happen.

Period sex might be the missing piece of the jigsaw in your relationship.

It can help you build trust and intimacy in your relationship.

Explore!!